Kegel Exercises for Women

Identifying the Need for Kegel Exercises

By

Emily Ambre

Table of Contents

CHAPTER 1

Introduction to Kegel Exercises

What are Kegel Exercises

Kegel exercises, also known as pelvic floor exercises, are a series of exercises that target and strengthen the pelvic floor muscles. The pelvic floor muscles are a group of muscles that support the organs in the pelvis, including the bladder, uterus, and rectum. These exercises were developed by Dr. Arnold Kegel, an American gynecologist, in the late 1940s to help women improve their pelvic floor muscle strength and treat various pelvic floor disorders.

Kegel exercises primarily involve contracting and relaxing the pelvic floor muscles. The exercises can be performed discreetly and are beneficial for both men and women, although they are more commonly associated with women's health. Kegel exercises are simple, convenient, and can be done at any age.

History of Kegel Exercises

Kegel exercises are named after Dr. Arnold Kegel, an American gynecologist who introduced them in the late 1940s. Dr. Kegel developed these exercises as a non-surgical alternative to treat urinary incontinence in women, particularly after childbirth. His initial research focused on identifying the role of the pelvic floor muscles in maintaining continence.

Dr. Kegel's pioneering work involved developing a device called the perineometer, which measured the strength of the pelvic floor muscles. He then prescribed specific exercises to strengthen these muscles based on the feedback provided by the device. Over time, the exercises became widely known as "Kegel exercises" in his honor.

Since their inception, Kegel exercises have gained recognition as an effective method for improving pelvic floor strength and managing various pelvic floor disorders. They have evolved to include different variations and techniques, and their benefits have been extensively studied and documented in the fields of urogynecology, obstetrics, physiotherapy, and sexual medicine.

Today, Kegel exercises are recommended by healthcare professionals worldwide as a first-line treatment for urinary incontinence and other pelvic floor-related issues. They are considered a safe, non-invasive, and cost-effective approach to improving pelvic floor muscle function.

In recent years, the awareness and importance of Kegel exercises have expanded beyond clinical settings. Many fitness and wellness programs now incorporate Kegel exercises to promote overall pelvic health and well-being. Additionally, with the rise of digital health and smartphone applications, there are now numerous apps and devices available that provide guidance and tracking for

Kegel exercises, making it easier for individuals to incorporate them into their daily routines.

Kegel exercises are a valuable tool for women (and men) to improve pelvic floor muscle strength and address various pelvic floor issues. With their rich history and proven benefits, Kegel exercises continue to play a crucial role in enhancing bladder control, sexual health, and overall pelvic well-being.

CHAPTER 2

Understanding the Pelvic Floor

Anatomy of the Pelvic Floor Muscles

The pelvic floor muscles are a complex network of muscles, ligaments, and connective tissues that span the bottom of the pelvis, providing support to the pelvic organs and playing a crucial role in various bodily functions. To truly understand the pelvic floor, it is essential to delve into the detailed anatomy of these muscles and their interconnected structure, here are some of the anatomy of the pelvic floor muscles:

1. Levator Ani Muscles: The levator ani muscles are the primary muscles of the pelvic floor and form a broad, hammock-like structure. They consist of bilateral muscle groups, with each side including the following three components:

1.1 Pubococcygeus (PC) Muscles: The pubococcygeus muscles, commonly referred to as the PC muscles, are the largest and most significant part of the levator ani. They extend from the pubic bone at the front of the pelvis to the coccyx (tailbone) at the back. The PC muscles form a U-shaped loop that surrounds the urethra, vagina, and rectum. These muscles play a vital role in maintaining continence, supporting the pelvic organs, and contributing to sexual function.

1.2 Puborectalis Muscle: The puborectalis muscle is a segment of the levator ani that wraps around the rectum in a sling-like fashion. It attaches to the pubic bone and merges with the other components of the levator ani. The puborectalis muscle assists in creating an angle in the rectum, aiding in the voluntary control of defecation.

1.3 Iliococcygeus Muscle: The iliococcygeus muscles are positioned behind the pubococcygeus muscles and extend from the ischial spine (a bony prominence in the pelvis) to the coccyx. These muscles provide support to the pelvic organs and help maintain the integrity of the pelvic floor.

2.Coccygeus Muscles: The coccygeus muscles, also known as the ischiococcygeus muscles, are located behind the levator ani muscles. They extend from the ischial spine to the coccyx and complete the posterior part of the pelvic floor. The coccygeus muscles contribute to the support and stability of the pelvic organs.

3. Perineal Muscles: The perineal muscles are located in the perineum, the region between the anus and the external genitalia. These muscles provide additional support to the pelvic floor and are crucial for urinary and fecal continence, sexual function, and stability of the pelvic floor. The key perineal muscles include:

3.1 Bulbocavernosus Muscle: The bulbocavernosus muscle surrounds the bulb of the penis in males or the vestibular bulbs in females. It plays a role in sexual function by aiding in erection and ejaculation in males and clitoral erection in females.

3.2 Superficial and Deep Transverse Perineal Muscles: The superficial and deep transverse perineal muscles are located in the perineum and contribute to the stability and support of the pelvic floor. They assist in maintaining continence and stabilizing the pelvic organs.

4. External Anal Sphincter Muscle: The external anal sphincter is a circular muscle that encircles the anus. It is under voluntary control and plays a crucial role in maintaining bowel continence. The external anal sphincter contracts to close the anus and relaxes to allow for bowel movements.

It's important to understand that the pelvic floor muscles are not isolated entities but are interconnected with other structures in the pelvis. They work in coordination with the deep abdominal muscles, hip muscles, and diaphragm to provide stability, support, and control to the pelvis.

The pelvic floor muscles are innervated by the pudendal nerve, which originates from the sacral nerve roots (S2-S4). The pudendal nerve supplies motor and sensory fibers to the pelvic floor muscles, allowing for voluntary control and sensation in the pelvic region.

Blood supply to the pelvic floor muscles is primarily derived from branches of the internal iliac arteries, including the inferior rectal arteries, vaginal arteries (in females), and the perineal artery. These arteries ensure an adequate oxygen and nutrient supply to the pelvic floor muscles for their proper functioning.

Understanding the intricate anatomy of the pelvic floor muscles is crucial in diagnosing and treating various pelvic floor disorders, such as urinary incontinence, pelvic organ prolapse, pelvic pain, and sexual dysfunction. Healthcare professionals specializing in pelvic health, such as gynecologists, urologists, and physiotherapists, utilize this knowledge to assess muscle function, perform pelvic floor muscle training, and guide interventions tailored to specific patient needs.

By comprehending the complex interplay of the pelvic floor muscles with other pelvic structures, individuals can develop a deeper understanding of the importance of maintaining the strength, coordination, and health of these muscles. This understanding serves as a foundation for targeted exercises like Kegel exercises and facilitates the prevention and management of pelvic floor disorders, leading to improved quality of life and overall well-being.

CHAPTER 3

Function of the Pelvic Floor Muscles

The pelvic floor muscles play a vital role in supporting the pelvic organs, maintaining continence, facilitating sexual function, and providing stability to the pelvis. Understanding the functions of the pelvic floor muscles is essential in comprehending their significance in overall health and well-being. Here are some functions of pelvic floor muscles:

1. Support of Pelvic Organs: The primary function of the pelvic floor muscles is to provide support to the pelvic organs,

including the bladder, uterus, and rectum. These muscles form a strong foundation, preventing the descent or prolapse of these organs. By maintaining the proper position and alignment of the pelvic organs, the pelvic floor muscles help prevent issues such as urinary incontinence and pelvic organ prolapse.

2. Control of Urinary Continence: The pelvic floor muscles play a crucial role in maintaining urinary continence. When the muscles are strong and functioning properly, they help keep the urethra closed, preventing the involuntary leakage of urine. The pelvic floor muscles contract to support the bladder and urethra

during activities that increase abdominal pressure, such as coughing, sneezing, laughing, or physical exertion, preventing urine leakage.

3. Bowel Control: In addition to urinary continence, the pelvic floor muscles contribute to bowel control. The muscles surrounding the rectum help maintain the integrity of the anal sphincter and rectal canal, allowing for voluntary control over bowel movements. The pelvic floor muscles contract to keep the anal sphincter closed, preventing involuntary passage of stool until it is appropriate to have a bowel movement.

4. Sexual Function: The pelvic floor muscles play a significant role in sexual function and

satisfaction for both men and women. In females, the muscles support the vaginal walls, contribute to vaginal tone, and assist in clitoral erection. In males, the pelvic floor muscles contribute to erectile function, ejaculation, and orgasmic intensity. Strong and coordinated pelvic floor muscles can enhance sexual arousal, improve orgasm quality, and provide greater sexual satisfaction.

5. Stability and Posture: The pelvic floor muscles work in conjunction with the deep abdominal muscles, hip muscles, and diaphragm to provide stability and support to the pelvis and spine. They form part of the core muscle group

and contribute to maintaining proper posture, body alignment, and spinal stability. The pelvic floor muscles work dynamically with these surrounding muscles during activities such as walking, running, lifting, and other functional movements.

6. Childbirth Support: During childbirth, the pelvic floor muscles undergo significant strain. They stretch and accommodate the passage of the baby through the birth canal. Strong and well-functioning pelvic floor muscles help support the weight of the baby and assist in the pushing phase of labor. After childbirth, the pelvic floor muscles play a crucial role in

postpartum recovery and restoration of pelvic floor function.

Understanding the multifaceted functions of the pelvic floor muscles highlights their significance in various aspects of health and well-being. Strong, flexible, and coordinated pelvic floor muscles are essential for maintaining continence, supporting pelvic organs, promoting sexual function, ensuring stability, and contributing to overall pelvic health. Regular exercise and targeted training, such as Kegel exercises, can help optimize the function of the pelvic floor muscles and prevent or manage pelvic floor disorders.

CHAPTER 4

Common Pelvic Floor Issues

The pelvic floor is a complex structure, and various factors can lead to dysfunction or disorders within this area. Understanding the common pelvic floor issues is essential for recognizing symptoms, seeking appropriate treatment, and maintaining pelvic health. Here are some of the most prevalent pelvic floor issues:

1. Urinary Incontinence: Urinary incontinence refers to the involuntary loss of urine, and it is a common pelvic floor issue, particularly among women.

There are different types of
urinary incontinence, including:

1.1 Stress Incontinence: Stress
incontinence occurs when there is
increased pressure on the bladder,
leading to urine leakage during
activities such as coughing, sneezing,
laughing, or physical exertion. Weak
pelvic floor muscles, compromised
urethral support, or damage to the
urinary sphincter can contribute to
stress incontinence.

1.2 Urge Incontinence: Urge
incontinence involves a sudden and
intense urge to urinate, followed by an
involuntary loss of urine. It can be
caused by an overactive bladder
muscle or abnormal nerve signals
between the bladder and the brain.

1.3 Mixed Incontinence: Mixed
incontinence refers to a combination

of stress and urge incontinence, where both symptoms are present.

2. Pelvic Organ Prolapse: Pelvic organ prolapse occurs when the pelvic organs, such as the bladder, uterus, or rectum, descend or protrude into the vaginal canal. Weakness or damage to the pelvic floor muscles and supporting tissues can result in pelvic organ prolapse. Symptoms may include a sensation of pelvic pressure or heaviness, a bulge or protrusion in the vaginal area, difficulties with bowel movements or urination, and discomfort during sexual intercourse.

3. Pelvic Floor Dysfunction: Pelvic floor dysfunction refers to a range of disorders that

affect the function of the pelvic floor muscles. It can involve muscle weakness, muscle tightness or hypertonicity, or coordination issues within the pelvic floor. Pelvic floor dysfunction may manifest as pelvic pain, discomfort, or difficulty with bladder or bowel control. It can be caused by various factors, including muscle imbalances, trauma, chronic tension, or neurological conditions.

4. Chronic Pelvic Pain: Chronic pelvic pain is persistent pain in the pelvic region lasting for at least six months. It can be caused by a variety of factors, such as pelvic floor muscle tension, nerve irritation, inflammation, or underlying

medical conditions. Chronic pelvic pain can significantly impact a person's quality of life, causing discomfort, distress, and affecting daily activities.

5. Sexual Dysfunction: Pelvic floor issues can contribute to sexual dysfunction in both men and women. For women, conditions such as pelvic organ prolapse, pelvic pain, or muscle weakness can lead to pain during intercourse (dyspareunia), reduced sexual satisfaction, or difficulties achieving orgasm. In men, pelvic floor dysfunction can result in erectile dysfunction, ejaculatory disorders, or discomfort in the genital or rectal area.

6. Postpartum Pelvic Floor Issues: Pregnancy and childbirth can place significant strain on the pelvic floor muscles, leading to various issues postpartum. These may include weakened pelvic floor muscles, urinary incontinence, pelvic organ prolapse, or perineal pain or trauma. Postpartum pelvic floor rehabilitation is crucial to support recovery and restore optimal pelvic floor function.

7. Male Pelvic Floor Issues: While pelvic floor issues are commonly associated with women, men can also experience pelvic floor dysfunction. Men may suffer from chronic pelvic pain, urinary symptoms, erectile dysfunction, or discomfort in

the genital or rectal area. These issues can be caused by muscle imbalances, trauma, prostate conditions, or other underlying factors.

Understanding the common pelvic floor issues is the first step towards addressing and managing them effectively. If you experience any symptoms related to urinary incontinence, pelvic organ prolapses, pelvic pain, sexual dysfunction, or other pelvic floor concerns, it is important to consult with a healthcare professional specializing in pelvic health. They can provide a thorough evaluation, offer appropriate treatment options, and guide you in pelvic floor exercises, such as Kegel exercises, that can help strengthen and rehabilitate the pelvic floor muscles. With proper diagnosis, treatment, and pelvic floor muscle training, many pelvic floor issues can be effectively managed, improving overall pelvic health and quality of life.

CHAPTER 5

Identifying the Need for Kegel Exercises

Signs of a Weak Pelvic Floor

A weak pelvic floor can lead to various issues and discomfort, affecting both men and women. Recognizing the signs of a weak pelvic floor is essential in identifying the need for exercises like Kegel exercises to strengthen these muscles. Here are some common signs and symptoms of a weak pelvic floor:

1. Urinary Incontinence: One of the primary signs of a weak pelvic floor is urinary incontinence, the involuntary leakage of urine. This can occur

during activities that increase abdominal pressure, such as coughing, sneezing, laughing, or physical exertion. Weak pelvic floor muscles may fail to provide adequate support to the bladder and urethra, leading to urine leakage. Stress incontinence, characterized by leakage during these activities, is a common indicator of a weak pelvic floor.

2. Frequency and Urgency: A weak pelvic floor can contribute to increased frequency and urgency of urination. You may feel the need to urinate more frequently throughout the day or experience a sudden, intense urge to urinate that is difficult to control. These symptoms can

be a result of compromised muscle strength and coordination within the pelvic floor.

3. Difficulty Controlling Bowel Movements: A weakened pelvic floor can impact bowel control, leading to difficulties in controlling bowel movements. You may experience fecal incontinence, which involves the involuntary leakage of stool or difficulty controlling gas. A weak pelvic floor can compromise the integrity of the anal sphincter muscles, making it challenging to maintain continence.

4. Pelvic Organ Prolapse: A significant sign of a weak pelvic floor is the development of pelvic organ prolapse. Pelvic

organ prolapse occurs when the pelvic organs, such as the bladder, uterus, or rectum, descend or protrude into the vaginal canal. Weakness or damage to the pelvic floor muscles and supporting tissues can contribute to this condition. Symptoms may include a sensation of pelvic pressure or heaviness, a bulge or protrusion in the vaginal area, difficulties with bowel movements or urination, and discomfort during sexual intercourse.

5. Decreased Sexual Satisfaction: A weak pelvic floor can negatively impact sexual function and satisfaction. In women, weakened pelvic floor muscles can result in reduced vaginal tone, decreased

sensation, and difficulties reaching orgasm. In men, it can contribute to erectile dysfunction or difficulties with ejaculation. Strengthening the pelvic floor muscles through exercises like Kegels can enhance sexual function and satisfaction.

6. Chronic Pelvic Pain: Chronic pelvic pain is a persistent discomfort in the pelvic region lasting for at least six months. Weakness or dysfunction of the pelvic floor muscles can contribute to pelvic pain. The pain may be dull or sharp, and it can vary in intensity and location. It may be present during specific activities or even at rest. Chronic pelvic pain can significantly impact a

person's quality of life, and addressing the underlying pelvic floor weakness is crucial in managing this condition.

7. Lower Back Pain and Postural Issues: A weak pelvic floor can affect the stability and alignment of the pelvis, leading to lower back pain and postural problems. The pelvic floor muscles work in conjunction with other core muscles to provide stability and support to the spine and pelvis. When the pelvic floor is weak, it can compromise the overall stability of the pelvis, contributing to lower back pain and difficulties with posture.

8. Difficulty during Pregnancy and Postpartum: During pregnancy and childbirth, the

pelvic floor muscles undergo significant strain. A weak pelvic floor can result in increased difficulties during pregnancy, such as urinary incontinence, pelvic pain, or pelvic organ prolapse. After childbirth, the pelvic floor muscles may remain weakened, leading to continued issues with urinary incontinence, pelvic organ support, or discomfort during the postpartum period. Strengthening the pelvic floor muscles through exercises like Kegels is crucial for the recovery and restoration of optimal pelvic floor function.

It's important to note that experiencing one or more of these signs does not necessarily mean that the pelvic floor muscles are weak.

However, if you consistently experience any of these symptoms or suspect a weak pelvic floor, it is recommended to consult with a healthcare professional specializing in pelvic health. They can assess your condition, provide a proper diagnosis, and recommend appropriate treatment options, which may include Kegel exercises or other targeted pelvic floor muscle training techniques.

Kegel exercises are specifically designed to strengthen the pelvic floor muscles. These exercises involve contracting and relaxing the muscles that control urinary and bowel function, thereby improving muscle tone, endurance, and coordination. Regular practice of Kegel exercises can help address the signs of a weak pelvic floor, improve bladder and bowel control, support pelvic organ health, enhance sexual function, and alleviate related symptoms.

A healthcare professional can guide you on the correct technique and progression of Kegel exercises tailored to your specific needs. They may recommend incorporating biofeedback devices, pelvic floor physical therapy, or other specialized interventions to optimize your pelvic floor muscle training.

Remember that consistency is key when performing Kegel exercises. By incorporating these exercises into your daily routine and gradually increasing the intensity and duration over time, you can effectively strengthen your pelvic floor muscles and improve their function, leading to better overall pelvic health and quality of life.

Factors Contributing to Pelvic Floor Weakness

Pelvic floor weakness can occur due to various factors, and recognizing these contributors is essential in identifying the need for exercises like Kegel exercises to strengthen the pelvic floor muscles. While both men and women can experience pelvic floor weakness, it is more commonly associated with women due to factors such as pregnancy, childbirth, and hormonal changes. These are some factors that can contribute to pelvic floor weakness:

1. Pregnancy and Childbirth: Pregnancy and childbirth can place significant strain on the pelvic floor muscles, leading to weakness. Factors that contribute to pelvic floor weakness during pregnancy

include hormonal changes, increased pressure on the pelvic floor due to the growing uterus, and stretching of the pelvic floor tissues to accommodate the developing baby. During vaginal delivery, the pelvic floor muscles undergo further stretching and may experience trauma or tears, weakening their integrity. Multiple pregnancies and prolonged pushing during labor can exacerbate the risk of pelvic floor weakness.

2. Aging: As we age, the pelvic floor muscles naturally lose strength and elasticity. The decline in estrogen levels during menopause can further contribute to pelvic floor weakness in women.

Additionally, hormonal changes associated with aging can affect tissue integrity, leading to decreased muscle tone and support within the pelvic floor.

3. Obesity: Excess weight and obesity can put additional strain on the pelvic floor muscles. The increased intra-abdominal pressure associated with obesity can weaken the pelvic floor over time. This pressure can contribute to urinary incontinence, pelvic organ prolapses, and other pelvic floor issues.

4. Chronic Constipation: Chronic constipation, characterized by infrequent bowel movements and difficulty passing stools, can strain the pelvic floor

muscles. Frequent straining during bowel movements puts pressure on the pelvic floor, leading to muscle fatigue and weakness over time.

5. Chronic Coughing: Persistent or chronic coughing, such as that caused by conditions like chronic bronchitis, asthma, or smoking, can also weaken the pelvic floor muscles. The repeated forceful contractions of the diaphragm and abdominal muscles during coughing can place stress on the pelvic floor, leading to muscle fatigue and decreased strength.

6. High-Impact Activities and Heavy Lifting: Engaging in high-impact activities such as running, jumping, or intense

weightlifting without proper pelvic floor muscle support and control can contribute to pelvic floor weakness. These activities create increased intra-abdominal pressure, which can strain the pelvic floor muscles if they are not adequately strong or coordinated.

7. Hormonal Changes: Hormonal fluctuations, particularly in women, can impact the strength and integrity of the pelvic floor muscles. Hormonal changes during the menstrual cycle, pregnancy, and menopause can affect tissue elasticity and overall muscle function, potentially leading to pelvic floor weakness.

8. Pelvic Surgeries: Certain surgical procedures, such as

hysterectomy (removal of the uterus), prostate surgery, or pelvic organ prolapse repair, can weaken the pelvic floor muscles. These surgeries may involve cutting or stretching the supportive tissues of the pelvic floor, potentially compromising muscle strength and function.

9. Sedentary Lifestyle: A sedentary lifestyle, characterized by prolonged periods of sitting or lack of regular physical activity, can contribute to pelvic floor weakness. Insufficient physical activity can lead to muscle deconditioning, including the pelvic floor muscles, resulting in decreased strength and control.

10. Genetic Factors and Connective Tissue Disorders: Some individuals may have a genetic predisposition to weaker connective tissues, including those within the pelvic floor. Certain connective tissue disorders, such as Ehlers-Danlos syndrome or Marfan syndrome, can affect the strength and integrity of pelvic floor tissues, potentially leading to weakness.

Identifying the factors contributing to pelvic floor weakness is crucial in understanding the need for exercises like Kegel exercises to strengthen the pelvic floor muscles. If you experience symptoms of a weak pelvic floor or identify any of these contributing factors, it is advisable to consult with a healthcare professional specializing in pelvic health. They can assess your condition, provide a proper diagnosis, and recommend appropriate treatment options, which may include pelvic floor exercises like Kegels.

Who Can Benefit from Kegel Exercises

Kegel exercises are a versatile and beneficial form of exercise for a wide range of individuals. While Kegel exercises are often associated with women, both men and women can benefit from incorporating these exercises into their routine. Identifying the need for Kegel exercises involves recognizing various conditions, stages of life, and circumstances where strengthening the pelvic floor muscles can be advantageous. Here are some benefit from Kegel exercises:

1. Women of All Ages: Women of all ages can benefit from Kegel exercises to strengthen their pelvic floor muscles. Regularly performing Kegel exercises can help prevent and manage various pelvic floor issues that women may experience throughout their lives, such as urinary incontinence, pelvic organ prolapse, pelvic pain, and sexual dysfunction. Kegel exercises are particularly beneficial during pregnancy and postpartum to support the pelvic floor and aid in recovery.

2. Pregnant Women: Pregnancy places increased strain on the pelvic floor muscles due to

hormonal changes, increased
pressure on the pelvic area, and
the stretching of tissues to
accommodate the growing
baby. Engaging in Kegel
exercises during pregnancy can
help strengthen the pelvic floor
muscles, support the weight of
the baby, improve bladder
control, and potentially reduce
the risk of urinary incontinence
and pelvic organ prolapse.
Kegel exercises during
pregnancy can also contribute
to a faster postpartum recovery.

3. Postpartum Women: After
   childbirth, the pelvic floor
   muscles may be weakened or
   stretched, leading to issues such
   as urinary incontinence, pelvic
   organ prolapse, or perineal
   pain. Kegel exercises are highly

beneficial for postpartum women as they can help restore strength and tone to the pelvic floor muscles, improve urinary and bowel control, support pelvic organ function, and promote healing in the perineal area. It is important to consult with a healthcare professional before starting Kegel exercises in the postpartum period to ensure proper technique and timing.

4. Women Experiencing Menopause: During menopause, hormonal changes can affect the strength and integrity of the pelvic floor muscles. Declining estrogen levels can lead to muscle atrophy, decreased tissue elasticity, and increased

vulnerability to pelvic floor issues. Regularly performing Kegel exercises during menopause can help maintain or improve the strength and tone of the pelvic floor muscles, reducing the risk of urinary incontinence, pelvic organ prolapses, and sexual dysfunction.

5. Men with Pelvic Floor Issues: While pelvic floor issues are commonly associated with women, men can also experience pelvic floor dysfunction and related issues. Men may suffer from urinary incontinence, erectile dysfunction, chronic pelvic pain, or discomfort in the genital or rectal area. Kegel exercises can be beneficial for

men with pelvic floor issues as they can help strengthen the pelvic floor muscles, improve bladder and bowel control, enhance erectile function, and alleviate pelvic pain.

6. Athletes and Active Individuals: Engaging in high-impact activities or intense physical training can put strain on the pelvic floor muscles. Athletes and active individuals, both men and women, can benefit from incorporating Kegel exercises into their training routine. Strengthening the pelvic floor muscles can provide better support to the pelvis, enhance stability, reduce the risk of pelvic floor dysfunction, and improve overall athletic performance.

7. Individuals with a Sedentary
   Lifestyle: Individuals with a
   sedentary lifestyle, such as
   those who spend prolonged
   periods sitting or have limited
   physical activity, can
   experience weakened pelvic
   floor muscles. Incorporating
   Kegel exercises into their daily
   routine can help strengthen the
   pelvic floor muscles, improve
   posture, and support bladder
   and bowel control.

8. Individuals Preparing for Pelvic
   Floor Surgery:

Individuals who are scheduled for or
considering pelvic floor surgery, such
as procedures for pelvic organ
prolapse or urinary incontinence, can
benefit from pre-surgical and post-
surgical pelvic floor muscle training.
Strengthening the pelvic floor

muscles before surgery can help optimize surgical outcomes, while post-surgical exercises, including Kegel exercises, can aid in recovery, promote healing, and enhance long-term results.

9. Individuals with Pelvic Floor Dysfunction or Pain: People experiencing pelvic floor dysfunction, including chronic pelvic pain, may find relief and improvement through targeted pelvic floor muscle exercises like Kegel exercises. Strengthening the pelvic floor muscles can help alleviate symptoms, enhance muscle coordination and control, reduce pain, and improve overall pelvic floor function.

10. Older Adults: As we age, the pelvic floor muscles naturally

lose strength and elasticity. Older adults, both men and women, can benefit from incorporating Kegel exercises into their routine to maintain or improve the strength and function of the pelvic floor muscles. Strengthening the pelvic floor can help prevent or manage urinary incontinence, support pelvic organ health, and improve overall quality of life in the senior population.

11. Prevention and Maintenance: Even in the absence of specific symptoms or conditions, incorporating Kegel exercises into one's routine as a preventive measure can be beneficial. Regularly performing Kegel exercises can help maintain the strength and

tone of the pelvic floor muscles, reduce the risk of future pelvic floor issues, and support overall pelvic health.

It is important to note that while Kegel exercises can be beneficial for many individuals, it is essential to perform them correctly and with guidance, particularly if you have specific pelvic floor issues or concerns. Consulting with a healthcare professional specializing in pelvic health, such as a gynecologist, urologist, or pelvic floor physical therapist, can provide personalized guidance, ensure proper technique, and tailor the exercises to your individual needs.

Kegel exercises offer numerous benefits for a wide range of individuals, including women of all ages, pregnant and postpartum women, men with pelvic floor issues, athletes, individuals with a sedentary lifestyle, those preparing for pelvic floor surgery, individuals with pelvic floor dysfunction or pain, older adults, and as a preventive measure. By strengthening the pelvic floor muscles through regular and correct practice of Kegel exercises, individuals can improve bladder and bowel control, support pelvic organ function, enhance sexual health, reduce the risk of pelvic floor issues, and promote overall pelvic well-being.

CHAPTER 6

Some Key Points to Consider when Incorporating Kegel Exercises

Kegel exercises specifically target and strengthen the pelvic floor muscles. By regularly performing Kegel exercises, you can improve muscle tone, endurance, and coordination within the pelvic floor, addressing the weakness and associated symptoms. Here are some key points to consider when incorporating Kegel exercises into your routine:

1. Correct Technique: It is important to learn and practice the correct technique of Kegel exercises to ensure optimal results. A healthcare professional, such as a physiotherapist or urologist, can provide guidance on how to correctly identify and isolate the pelvic floor muscles and guide you through the exercise technique.

2. Consistency and Gradual Progression: Like any exercise, consistency is key. Regularly performing Kegel exercises, ideally on a daily basis, is important to see improvements in pelvic floor strength. Start with a comfortable number of repetitions and gradually increase the intensity and

duration of the exercises over time. It's important to progress gradually to avoid overexertion or muscle fatigue.

3. Incorporating Functional Movements: While Kegel exercises are primarily focused on isolating the pelvic floor muscles, it is also important to incorporate functional movements into your exercise routine. Functional movements, such as squats and bridges, engage the entire core and lower body, including the pelvic floor muscles. Integrating these movements can help strengthen the pelvic floor muscles in a functional context.

4. Biofeedback and Pelvic Floor Rehabilitation Devices:

Biofeedback devices or pelvic floor rehabilitation devices can assist in the proper performance of Kegel exercises. These devices provide real-time feedback on muscle contractions, helping you identify and engage the correct muscles. They can be particularly useful for individuals who have difficulty isolating the pelvic floor muscles or need assistance in monitoring progress.

5. Comprehensive Pelvic Floor Rehabilitation: In some cases, a comprehensive pelvic floor rehabilitation program may be recommended. This may involve working with a pelvic floor physical therapist who can

provide specialized exercises, manual therapy techniques, and additional treatments tailored to your specific needs. They can address any underlying muscle imbalances, coordination issues, or related conditions contributing to pelvic floor weakness.

By recognizing the factors that contribute to pelvic floor weakness and incorporating appropriate exercises like Kegel exercises into your routine, you can strengthen the pelvic floor muscles and improve their function. It is important to seek guidance from a healthcare professional to ensure proper technique and personalized recommendations based on your unique circumstances. Strengthening the pelvic floor can help alleviate symptoms, improve pelvic organ support, enhance urinary and bowel control, and promote overall pelvic health and well-being.

CHAPTER 7

How to Perform Kegel Exercises

Locating the Pelvic Floor Muscles

Before delving into the instructions for performing Kegel exercises, it is crucial to understand how to correctly locate the pelvic floor muscles. The pelvic floor muscles are a group of muscles located at the bottom of the pelvis, extending from the pubic bone at the front to the tailbone at the back. Identifying and isolating these muscles is essential to ensure the effectiveness of Kegel exercises. Here are some steps to help you locate the pelvic floor muscles:

1. Relax and Find a Comfortable Position: Begin by finding a comfortable position to perform the exercise. You can choose to sit, stand, or lie down. It's important to relax your body and take slow, deep breaths to promote a relaxed state.

2. Identify the Pelvic Floor Muscles: To identify the pelvic floor muscles, imagine that you are trying to stop the flow of urine midstream. It's important to note that this is only an exercise to identify the muscles and should not be done regularly during urination, as it can disrupt the normal emptying of the bladder. Try to

contract the muscles around the urethra and anus without squeezing the buttocks or thighs. The feeling is often described as a gentle lifting or squeezing sensation.

3. Visualize the Muscles: If you are having difficulty identifying the pelvic floor muscles, you can try visualizing the muscles involved. Imagine that you are sitting on a marble and want to lift it up using only your pelvic floor muscles. Visualizing this lifting action can help you connect with the correct muscles.

4. Engage Only the Pelvic Floor Muscles: It's essential to ensure that you are isolating and engaging only the pelvic floor muscles without involving

other muscles in the abdomen, buttocks, or thighs. Take care not to hold your breath while performing the exercise. It is recommended to continue breathing naturally throughout the exercise.

5. Seek Professional Guidance if Needed: If you are having difficulty locating the pelvic floor muscles or are unsure if you are performing the exercise correctly, seeking guidance from a healthcare professional specializing in pelvic health, such as a pelvic floor physical therapist, can be beneficial. They can provide personalized instruction, perform an assessment, and guide you in proper technique and muscle activation.

It's important to note that Kegel exercises may not be suitable or effective for everyone. Some individuals may require a more comprehensive pelvic floor rehabilitation program or specialized interventions tailored to their specific needs. Consulting with a healthcare professional specializing in pelvic health is recommended to ensure proper technique, personalized guidance, and individualized treatment.

Locating the pelvic floor muscles is a crucial first step in performing Kegel exercises effectively. By understanding the correct technique and engaging the pelvic floor muscles properly, you can maximize the benefits of these exercises. Remember to be patient, consistent, and seek professional guidance if needed. Strengthening the pelvic floor muscles through Kegel exercises can improve bladder and bowel control, support pelvic organ function, enhance sexual health, and promote overall pelvic well-being.

Step-by-Step Guide to Kegel Exercises

Performing Kegel exercises involves a series of steps to ensure proper technique and maximize effectiveness. Here is a step-by-step guide to performing Kegel exercises:

1. Find a Comfortable Position: Start by finding a comfortable position to perform the exercises. You can choose to sit, stand, or lie down. It's important to relax your body

and maintain good posture throughout the exercise.

2. Locate the Pelvic Floor Muscles: Identify and locate the pelvic floor muscles using the techniques mentioned earlier in this response. Focus on engaging only the pelvic floor muscles without involving other muscle groups.

3. Start with Relaxation: Begin with a relaxation phase to prepare the muscles. Take a few deep breaths and consciously relax your pelvic floor muscles.

4. Contract the Pelvic Floor Muscles: Once you are in a relaxed state, contract your pelvic floor muscles by squeezing and lifting them

upward and inward. Imagine pulling the muscles up as if you are trying to lift them towards your belly button. The contraction should be firm but not overly intense.

5. Hold the Contraction: Maintain the contraction of the pelvic floor muscles for a few seconds. Initially, aim for holding the contraction for 3-5 seconds. As you progress, you can gradually increase the duration up to 10 seconds or as recommended by a healthcare professional.

6. Relax and Rest: After holding the contraction, release the pelvic floor muscles and allow them to relax completely. Take a brief rest period before proceeding to the next

repetition. This relaxation phase is as important as the contraction phase.

7. Repeat the Exercise: Repeat the contraction and relaxation sequence for the desired number of repetitions. Start with a manageable number, such as 10 repetitions, and gradually increase over time as your muscles become stronger.

8. Establish a Routine: To experience the benefits of Kegel exercises, consistency is key. Establish a regular routine by performing the exercises at least three times a day. You can incorporate them into your daily schedule, such as during morning, afternoon, and evening routines, to ensure consistency.

Tips for Effective Kegel Exercises

To enhance the effectiveness of your Kegel exercises, here are some helpful tips:

1. Stay Focused: During the exercises, maintain focus on the pelvic floor muscles. Avoid distractions and concentrate on engaging and contracting the correct muscles.

2. Breathe Naturally: It is important to breathe naturally throughout the exercises. Avoid holding your breath, as it can create unnecessary tension in the body. Inhale deeply as you prepare for the contraction, and exhale as you release and relax the muscles.

3. Gradually Increase Intensity: As your pelvic floor muscles become stronger, you can gradually increase the intensity of the contractions. Start with gentle contractions and progress to stronger contractions over time. However, avoid straining or overexerting the muscles, as it can lead to discomfort or muscle fatigue.

4. Avoid Overuse of Abdominal or Buttock Muscles: Ensure that you are isolating the pelvic floor muscles during the exercises. Avoid excessive engagement of the abdominal or buttock muscles, as it can divert the focus from the pelvic floor muscles and reduce the effectiveness of the exercise.

5. Be Patient: Results from Kegel
    exercises may take time. It is
    important to be patient and
    persistent in your practice. It
    may take several weeks or even
    months of regular exercise to
    notice significant
    improvements in pelvic floor
    strength and function.

6. Seek Professional Guidance: If
    you are unsure about the
    technique or have specific
    pelvic floor concerns, seek
    guidance from a healthcare
    professional specializing in
    pelvic health. They can provide
    personalized instruction, assess
    your condition, and offer
    additional treatment options or
    modifications to optimize your
    pelvicfloor exercise routine.

7. Combine with Other Activities:
    Incorporate Kegel exercises
    into your daily routine by
    associating them with other
    activities. For example, you can
    perform Kegels while brushing
    your teeth, waiting in line, or
    during a specific daily ritual.
    This helps to establish a
    consistent habit and ensures
    that you do not forget to
    perform the exercises.

8. Use Biofeedback Devices:
    Consider using biofeedback
    devices or mobile apps
    designed to provide real-time
    feedback on your pelvic floor
    muscle contractions. These
    tools can help you monitor your
    progress, ensure proper
    technique, and motivate you to

stay consistent with your
exercises.

9. Modify as Needed: Individuals
have different levels of pelvic
floor strength and may require
modifications to the exercises.
If you find it challenging to
perform the exercises correctly
or experience discomfort,
consult with a healthcare
professional for guidance and
potential modifications tailored
to your needs.

10. Maintain Overall Pelvic Health:
In addition to Kegel exercises,
maintaining overall pelvic
health is important. Stay
hydrated, maintain a balanced
diet, practice good bowel
habits, and avoid activities that
put unnecessary strain on the
pelvic floor muscles. A holistic

approach to pelvic health can complement the benefits of Kegel exercises.

Remember, Kegel exercises are not a one-size-fits-all solution. It is important to customize the exercises based on your individual needs, consult with a healthcare professional, and adapt the routine as necessary. By following these step-by-step instructions and incorporating these tips, you can perform Kegel exercises effectively, improve the strength and function of your pelvic floor muscles, and promote overall pelvic health and well-being.

CHAPTER 8

Benefit of Kegel Exercises for Women

Kegel exercises offer numerous benefits for women by specifically targeting and strengthening the pelvic floor muscles. Here are some key benefits of Kegel exercises:

1. Improved Bladder Control: One of the primary benefits of Kegel exercises is improved bladder control. Strengthening the pelvic floor muscles helps to support the bladder and urethra, reducing the risk of urinary incontinence. Kegel exercises can be particularly beneficial for women who experience

stress incontinence, which is the leakage of urine during activities that put pressure on the bladder, such as coughing, sneezing, laughing, or exercising.

2. Treatment and Prevention of Urinary Incontinence: Kegel exercises are often recommended as a first-line treatment for various types of urinary incontinence in women. By strengthening the pelvic floor muscles, Kegel exercises can help manage and reduce the frequency and severity of urinary incontinence episodes.

3. Management of Pelvic Organ Prolapse: Pelvic organ prolapse occurs when the pelvic organs, such as the bladder, uterus, or rectum, descend or protrude

into the vaginal canal. Kegel exercises can help strengthen the pelvic floor muscles, providing better support for the pelvic organs and potentially slowing down the progression of pelvic organ prolapse. Kegels may also be part of the overall treatment plan for managing mild to moderate cases of pelvic organ prolapse.

4. Postpartum Recovery: Pregnancy and childbirth can significantly impact the pelvic floor muscles. Engaging in Kegel exercises during the postpartum period can aid in the recovery and restoration of pelvic floor strength and function. These exercises can help improve bladder control, promote healing in the perineal

area, and reduce the risk of urinary incontinence and pelvic organ prolapse following childbirth.

5. Enhanced Sexual Health: Strong pelvic floor muscles play a vital role in sexual health and satisfaction. By improving muscle tone and control, Kegel exercises can enhance vaginal muscle strength, increase sensitivity, and improve orgasmic potential. Additionally, stronger pelvic floor muscles can provide a greater sense of tightness during intercourse, potentially benefiting both the woman and her partner.

6. Prevention of Bowel Incontinence: Kegel exercises can also help prevent or

manage bowel incontinence. By strengthening the pelvic floor muscles, these exercises can improve control over the anal sphincter, reducing the risk of involuntary bowel movements or difficulty controlling gas.

7. Support During Menopause: Menopause is associated with hormonal changes that can weaken the pelvic floor muscles and lead to urinary incontinence, pelvic organ prolapse, and sexual dysfunction. Regularly performing Kegel exercises can help counteract the effects of hormonal changes, maintain pelvic floor strength, and manage or prevent these issues.

8. Improved Recovery After Gynecological Surgeries:

Women who undergo gynecological surgeries, such as hysterectomy or pelvic organ prolapse repair, can benefit from pre- and post-operative pelvic floor muscle training, including Kegel exercises. Strengthening the pelvic floor muscles before surgery can help optimize surgical outcomes, while exercises post-surgery can aid in recovery, reduce complications, and support long-term results.

9. Enhanced Core Stability: The pelvic floor muscles are an integral part of the core muscles, working in conjunction with the abdominal and back muscles. By strengthening the pelvic floor, Kegel exercises contribute to

overall core stability, which can improve posture, reduce lower back pain, and enhance overall body strength.

10. Improved Quality of Life: Strengthening the pelvic floor muscles through Kegel exercises can significantly improve the quality of life for women. By reducing or eliminating symptoms of urinary incontinence, pelvic organ prolapses, and sexual dysfunction, women can feel more confident, comfortable, and empowered in their daily activities and intimate relationships.

Kegel exercises offer numerous benefits for women, including improved bladder control, treatment and prevention of urinary

incontinence, management of pelvic
organ prolapse, postpartum recovery,
enhanced sexual health, prevention of
bowel incontinence, support during
menopause, improved recovery after
gynecological surgeries, enhanced
core stability, and an overall
improved quality of life.
Incorporating Kegel exercises into a
regular routine can help strengthen the
pelvic floor muscles, promote pelvic
health, and provide women with
greater control, comfort, and
confidence in various aspects of their
lives.